EMPATHIC

BIRTH-HER

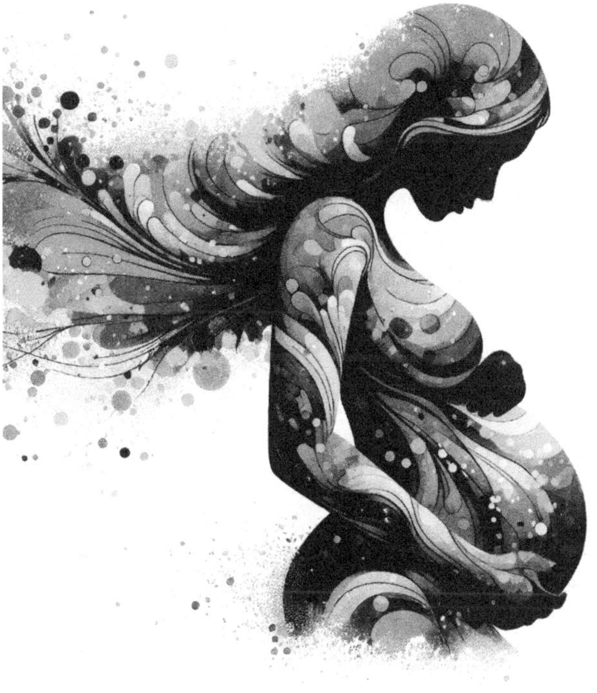

Felicia Francis-Edwards

Foreword
Dr. Candace Kelly

Empathic Birth-her: A Gentle Approach for Doulas in Birth and Beyond
by Felicia Edwards

Printed and bound in the United States of America

Published by Cole Publishing

Library of Congress
Cataloging-in-Publication Data
ISBN: 979-8-9918058-0-3

Cole Publishing
4067 Hardwick Street #282
Lakewood, CA 90712

Email: ccpprod@aol.com
Book Cover Design by Cole Publishing Graphic Team
For Book Orders:
Contact us at Cole Publishing Company
Contact us at Cole Publishing Company
www.ColePublishing.org
email: colepublishing2000@gmail.com

Cole Publishing

CONTENTS

DEDICATION

To the mothers and families who have allowed me to walk beside them during the most sacred moments of life—your trust and courage have inspired every word of this book.

To my fellow doulas, whose gentle strength and unwavering support continue to bring light and hope into the world—I am honored to stand among you as we guide each new beginning together.

And to my family, whose love has been my foundation—thank you for nurturing my spirit so that I may nurture others.

With gratitude and love,
Felicia

ACKNOWLEDGMENTS

To my husband, Brian Edwards: Your unwavering support has made my work as a doula not just possible, but durable. You've covered me in every way, lifting me up when I needed it most, and for that, I am forever grateful. You've given me the strength to be a "super doula," and it is with a smile on my face that I say thank you. I could not have done it without your steadfast love and encouragement. Thank you for praying for me, for interceding on my behalf, and for caring for me after those long, exhausting nights. "Thank you" doesn't even begin to express the depth of my gratitude. God placed you in my life for a purpose, and I am so blessed to have you by my side. Your constant support, love, and encouragement have been a blessing throughout this journey. I could not have done this without you by my side.

To my daughter, Simone Edwards: As my firstborn, you were an essential part of this journey. Your honest observations, encouraging words, and unwavering support helped me transition into this work. You spoke into my life, seeing the person I would become long before I did, and for that, I thank you. Your insight and wisdom have been invaluable, and I am deeply grateful for your love and belief in me.

To Kim Evans: Your support and empowerment on this journey of life have meant more to me than words can express. You have been a true champion for me, an encourager, and a motivator, always led by the Spirit of God. I've known you for a long time, and through all the highs and lows, you've consistently seen possibility when I was at my lowest. Thank you for co-laboring with me, for believing in me, and for walking with me to this very moment.

To my mom, Charliemae Frances: You encouraged me, affirmed me, loved on me, and trusted me in ways that shaped who I am today. Thank you for believing in me. As a mother of eight, you demonstrated tenacity, mental toughness, resilience, and, most importantly, a faith walk that has left a lasting imprint on my heart. I miss you so much, but I carry your strength and love with me every day. I will love and miss you forever.

To Cole Publishing: Thank you for your professionalism and your support. Your commitment to excellence and integrity is super amazing. Thank you for bringing this project to fruition. Your dedication and your effort are greatly appreciated.

To Dr. Candace Kelly: You have been my doula in more ways than one, sitting with me patiently, speaking into my life, being my Mordecai, and encouraging me even when I missed deadlines. With your soft, reassuring words—"Come on, sis, you can do this"—you never gave up on me. I marvel at your influence and boldness, and my heart's desire is to walk in that same strength for myself. Thank you for being such an inspiring role model, constantly reminding me that I can do all things through Christ who strengthens me. You always pushed me to keep going—chin to my chest—and PUSH!

FOREWORD

Rev. Dr. Candace Kelly

Doulas play an essential role in improving maternal health outcomes, particularly for women of color who face systemic disparities in healthcare. The presence of a doula—an advocate, support person, and educator—has been proven to enhance birth experiences, promote positive health outcomes, and contribute to closing the gap in maternal health disparities.

Advocacy and Support for Vulnerable Populations

It is historically know that women of color, particularly Black women, face higher risks of maternal mortality and morbidity compared to their white counterparts. The Centers for Disease Control and Prevention (CDC) reports that Black women are three to four times more likely to die from pregnancy-related complications. These disparities are often due to implicit biases in healthcare, lack of access to quality care, and systemic inequities.

Doulas act as a bridge between the healthcare system and their clients, providing a consistent source of support and advocacy. They ensure that birthing individuals' concerns are heard and respected, helping to navigate medical terminology, advocate for their clients' preferences, and intervene if necessary to ensure that care is delivered safely and respectfully. By advocating for clients, doulas help reduce the risk of medical interventions that may not be necessary, thereby improving health outcomes.

Closing the Disparities Gap

Doulas are uniquely positioned to address the disparities that exist in maternal healthcare. For communities of color, cultural competence in care is crucial. Doulas often come from similar backgrounds and can relate to their clients' experiences, fostering trust and communication. This familiarity enables doulas to offer culturally relevant support, empowering women to advocate for themselves and make informed decisions throughout pregnancy, labor, and postpartum.

Studies have shown that the continuous presence of a doula significantly reduces the likelihood of medical interventions such as cesarean sections, which are more common in women of color and can lead to further complications. Women who receive doula care are also less likely to experience preterm birth, which is a major contributor to infant mortality. This reduction in interventions and complications helps close the gap between women of color and their white counterparts in terms of health outcomes.

Reducing Stress and Improving Mental Health

Pregnancy and childbirth can be a vulnerable time for any woman, but for women of color facing racial bias, economic challenges, and limited access to healthcare, the stress can be overwhelming. This stress is associated with negative birth outcomes, including preterm labor and low birth weight. Doulas provide emotional support throughout the birthing process, helping to alleviate the stress of pregnancy and childbirth.

By offering a compassionate calming presence, teaching relaxation techniques, and providing continuous encouragement, doulas help improve the mental health of their clients. This emotional support reduces anxiety and empowers women to face labor with confidence. The impact of this support extends beyond the delivery room, as studies have shown that women who have the support of a doula are less likely to experience postpartum depression.

Education and Empowerment - One of the key roles of a doula is to provide education, which is crucial for birthing women, especially those who may not have had access to adequate prenatal care or health education. Doulas offer guidance on nutrition, prenatal care, and preparation for labor, as well as breastfeeding support and postpartum care.

For women who may have experienced neglect or marginalization in healthcare, this education is vital in empowering them to take control of their birthing experience. When women are informed about their bodies, the birth process, and their options, they are more likely to feel empowered to make decisions that lead to healthier outcomes for themselves and their babies.

Lowering Rates of Medical Interventions - Research has shown that women supported by doulas are less likely to require medical interventions such as epidurals, forceps, vacuum extraction, and cesarean sections. These interventions, while sometimes necessary, can increase the risk of complications for both the mother and the baby. By reducing the need for these interventions, doulas contribute to safer births and better health outcomes. For example, the continuous support provided by doulas helps to shorten labor, reduce the need for pain relief, and increase the likelihood of spontaneous vaginal delivery. This support also leads to higher satisfaction with the birth experience, which is linked to better mental and physical health in the postpartum period.

Building Trust in the Healthcare System - In communities where mistrust of the healthcare system runs deep due to historical and ongoing discrimination, doulas play a crucial role in rebuilding trust. A doula's presence can reassure clients that they are not alone in the healthcare system and that their voices will be heard. This trust-building is especially important for women of color who may have experienced trauma or disrespect in medical settings.

By providing a consistent, supportive presence, doulas help rebuild this trust, encouraging more women to seek prenatal care and to engage with the healthcare system in a positive way. Over time, this can lead to improved maternal and infant health outcomes across communities that have historically been underserved.

Doulas are more than just birth companions—they are advocates, educators, and champions for equitable maternal care. Their role in providing continuous emotional, physical, and informational support is critical in improving maternal outcomes, reducing health disparities, and ultimately saving lives. As we strive to create a more equitable healthcare system, particularly for Black women and other women of color, doulas remain a vital part of the solution. Their presence ensures that every mother, regardless of race or socioeconomic status, receives the respect, care, and support she deserves during one of the most significant moments of her life.

As a birthing professional, Felicia understands that birth is not just a medical event, but an emotional, spiritual, and transformative journey. With each mother she has served, Felicia has been more than a guide through labor and delivery—she has been an empathic and compassionate witness to the strength and resilience of women who deserve to be heard, supported, and treated with the utmost dignity.

In a world where disparities in maternal health care disproportionately affect women of color, Felicia's work has been a beacon of hope and a testament to the power of advocacy and education. Her unique ability to offer comfort, education, and an unwavering presence to her clients is a reflection of her deep empathy and understanding of the challenges many women face during childbirth.

Felicia's commitment to equitable maternal care goes beyond individual births. Through her leadership with Still Resilient Redefining Maternal and Infant Health, she has worked tirelessly to provide empathy-based education and training to hospitals, institutions, and birth workers, ensuring that more professionals understand the vital need for respectful and culturally competent care.

It is my hope that Felicia's book, her vision, and her unwavering dedication to the women she serves will inspire more doulas, healthcare providers, and advocates to step forward in the fight for equitable, safe, and respectful birthing experiences for all women. Every mother deserves the right to be seen, heard, and honored in the process of bringing new life into the world, and Felicia Edwards has dedicated her life to making that vision a reality.

PREFACE

Empathic birthing is a holistic approach to childbirth that emphasizes emotional connection, compassion, and understanding throughout the process of labor and delivery. It focuses on the emotional and psychological well-being of the mother, her partner, and the newborn, creating a nurturing and supportive environment.

Key aspects of empathic birthing include:

Emotional Support: Encouraging the presence of people who provide emotional comfort and reassurance, such as a partner, doula, or family members.

Active Listening: Caregivers (e.g., doctors, nurses, midwives) who focus on listening to the mother's needs, concerns, and desires, ensuring her voice is heard and respected in decision-making.

Mind-Body Connection: Incorporating relaxation techniques such as deep breathing, visualization, mindfulness, and meditation to help manage pain and anxiety.

Trauma-Informed Care: Recognizing past trauma and tailoring the birthing experience to avoid triggers, ensure safety, and foster empowerment.

Gentle Birthing Environment: Creating a calm, peaceful space with dim lighting, soothing music, or other personal preferences to minimize stress.

Birth Plans with Flexibility: Supporting the mother's birth plan while allowing room for flexibility if circumstances change, ensuring she feels in control and confident throughout the process.

Empathic birthing aims to foster a positive birth experience, improving the emotional bond between mother and child while enhancing the overall well-being of both. It can be especially beneficial for women who have had previous traumatic births or experiences with medical care.

Felicia Francis-Edwards

CHAPTER 1

An Urban Character

I still remember that first call, my phone buzzing in the middle of the night. It was Rochelle, my client. She'd been admitted to the hospital for an induction. "Alright," I told myself, "Here we go."

When I arrived, I could see the relief wash over her face, like someone had just turned the lights back on. She smiled, though I could tell she had the weight of the world on her shoulders. Rochelle was a 41-year-old mother of one, a brown-skinned, plus-sized woman facing more than her share of challenges. This induction wasn't just a medical procedure; it was layered with complexities—gestational diabetes, pregnancy-induced hypertension, and a high-risk pregnancy due to her age and health conditions. But that wasn't all.

You see, she was unhoused, fresh out of a program for pregnant and parenting women. There was no home waiting for her after this baby was born, just the unknown. Sitting there, I could feel her fears floating in the room like heavy fog—about the baby, about her future, about what lay ahead once those hospital doors opened and she had to walk out with a newborn in her arms but nowhere to go.

The induction itself was textbook—at least on the outside. She progressed well, dilating and effacing at a steady pace. There were a few heart rate dips with the baby, but nothing alarming. Still, Rochelle barely spoke as she labored. Silence is a language all its own, and hers was thick with unspoken words.

It wasn't long before she opened up. She told me she had to check into the hospital under an alias. Now, this caught me off guard. I mean, who expects to show up for a birth and suddenly feel like they're in a spy movie? Turns out, the father of her baby wasn't exactly winning any "Man of the Year" awards. From the moment she told him she was pregnant, he'd been pushing for her to have an abortion. When she stood her ground, he stormed out of her life, leaving behind only his anger and a heap of unresolved issues. She hadn't seen him since.

Fast forward to the day of the induction—Rochelle, in a moment of vulnerability, gave him a call. She told him what was happening, that she was about to bring his child into the world. But instead of offering support or even a lukewarm "good luck," he went off. He threatened her. Threatened her at a time when she needed love, support, and at least a decent apology. That's why she used the alias, to protect herself from someone who should've been protecting her.

The sadness in the room was overwhelming, like a third presence hovering between us. The sadness of a mother about to welcome a baby into a world of uncertainty, with no stable home, no supportive partner, and no clear path ahead. But despite all of that, she was brave. There she was, fighting through labor while carrying the weight of her circumstances—and still smiling when she saw me walk through that door.

In those quiet moments between contractions, I couldn't help but feel the enormity of her struggle. It was more than just physical pain. It was emotional, spiritual, the kind of weight that makes your bones ache. And yet, here she was, ready to bring a new life into the world. Despite everything, she pushed through. Because that's what mothers do, right? They push.

But let me tell you, if there was ever a time I felt the power of being a doula, it was in that hospital room with Rochelle. Her story wasn't unique, but it was hers, and I was there to witness her strength firsthand.

After four hours of labor, Rochelle was 6 cm dilated. The clock struck 7 PM, marking the beginning of the shift change. In Labor and Delivery, nurses work 12-hour shifts, and as the outgoing nurse prepared to hand over her responsibilities, I sensed a shift in the atmosphere. During shift changes, the nurse gives the incoming staff a report on the patient's condition and concerns, a critical moment in patient care.

While I stayed by Rochelle's side, the nurse was in and out of the room, checking the fetal monitor, adjusting leads, and assessing her vital signs. She was professional and helpful, but there was little interaction between them—no warmth, no personal connection. I couldn't help but notice this lack of bonding, and it made me uneasy.

As a doula, I've learned to be attuned to the nuances of patient care, and what I saw was disheartening. It often appears that non-Black nurses display their biases and prejudices toward Black women, sometimes unconsciously. It's the little things—like the failure to make eye contact, the omission of her name when addressing her, and the lack of explanations for the procedures being performed.

Here was a plus-sized woman over forty, unhoused, navigating a difficult labor, and dealing with conflict with the baby's father. Yet, somehow, she was not treated as if she mattered.

It became painfully clear that Rochelle was not the "ideal" patient in the eyes of the medical staff—not because of how she acted or spoke; for the most part, she remained quiet. But when she did voice her concerns, she may have come off as rough around the edges, and I couldn't shake the feeling that her appearance—a reflection of her struggles—led to her being perceived through a lens that skewed the reality of who she was. The stereotype of the "angry Black woman" seemed to loom over her like a dark cloud, influencing how the nurse interacted with her.

As the outgoing nurse transitioned to the incoming one, she gave a detailed report. They discussed Rochelle's progress, her medical conditions, and the necessary interventions for her care. On the surface, this sounds acceptable, right? A standard procedure in the hospital setting. But beneath the clinical jargon, I could sense an underlying narrative being spun. It felt as if the nurses were more focused on the challenges presented by Rochelle's situation rather than her strengths.

I watched them exchange glances, a mix of concern and judgment. My heart ached for Rochelle, who, despite her circumstances, was fighting for her baby and for herself. This was not just a labor and delivery; it was a human experience, a significant life event marred by societal biases that sought to overshadow her bravery and resilience.

As the new nurse stepped into the room, I made it my mission to advocate for Rochelle, to ensure she felt seen and heard amidst the clinical chatter. I gently squeezed her hand and offered reassuring words, reminding her that she was strong and deserving of the best care. In that moment, I knew that as her doula, my role extended far beyond just supporting her through labor; it was about ensuring her dignity was upheld, her voice amplified, and her humanity recognized.

This was the essence of my journey as a doula—a commitment to champion the women who often go unheard and unvalued. I couldn't change the system overnight, but I could be a source of support for Rochelle in her time of need. Together, we would navigate this experience, defying the biases that sought to diminish her spirit.

But there was a problem. The nurse was literally standing over Rochelle's head while giving the report, her body language closed off and focused on the incoming nurse.

They exchanged medical jargon, discussing my client's care as if she were a piece of furniture rather than a human being experiencing a pivotal moment in her life. I watched Rochelle's face closely; concern and puzzlement flickered across her features, but she remained silent. I could see the pain of being ignored etched in her expression, the questions swirling in her mind left unanswered.

As a doula, I knew precisely what I was witnessing. I saw this client being treated like she didn't matter, and it broke my heart. Neither nurse engaged her during the approximately 15 minutes they spoke, leaving her in the dark about what was happening with her own body. I could no longer remain silent; I had to say something.

I took a deep breath, summoning my courage, and approached the nurses. "Excuse me," I began, trying to keep my tone calm but firm. "I don't think it's appropriate for you to discuss my client's care without addressing her directly. She deserves to know what's going on." I gestured toward Rochelle. "Can you please explain her situation to her? She needs to be part of this conversation."

The nurses paused, glancing at each other, a hint of confusion in their eyes. They didn't seem to realize how their behavior had sidelined Rochelle, treating her like a bystander in her own experience. I turned back to my client, offering her a reassuring smile. "You're not invisible, and your voice matters," I whispered.

"Um, yes, of course," the outgoing nurse said, suddenly aware of the oversight. "I'm so sorry. We were just going over some information. Let's talk to you about everything."

They turned to Rochelle, finally engaging her in a way they should have done from the start. "So, just to fill you in, it's shift change right now," the incoming nurse said gently. "We wanted to update each other on your progress, but we should have included you. How are you feeling?"

Rochelle looked taken aback, as if she had just been pulled from a dream. "I—uh, I didn't know what was happening," she admitted, her voice barely above a whisper.

The nurses immediately began explaining the induction process, addressing her concerns and answering the questions she hadn't felt comfortable voicing earlier. It was a small step, but a crucial one. The tension in the room began to lift, and I could see Rochelle relax just a fraction as she became more involved in her care.

The nurses were apologetic, realizing their misstep. I could sense their genuine intent to do better; it just hadn't occurred to them that their approach was problematic. It drove home the stark reality of the situation: this client was perceived to be invisible, a person who didn't matter.

As the conversation shifted to include Rochelle, I felt a sense of relief wash over me. Advocacy was a vital part of my role, but it was also a reminder of how important it is to ensure every woman feels seen and heard, especially in vulnerable moments like these. I wanted Rochelle to know that she was not alone in this journey—that I was there to support her every step of the way.

This was a lesson for all of us, a reminder that in a healthcare setting, it's easy to forget the humanity of those we serve. Each patient has a story, a life filled with struggles and triumphs, and they deserve the respect and dignity that comes with being part of their own care. As the nurses continued to engage with Rochelle, I felt a renewed sense of purpose. This was why I had chosen this path: to advocate for women like her, to remind them of their worth, and to help them navigate the complexities of bringing new life into the world.

Seeing the look on Rochelle's face as the nurses spoke about her in her presence broke my heart. It was like watching someone be erased right before my eyes. They didn't know the complexities of her life—the dynamics that weighed heavily on her shoulders. They didn't know that she was just weeks away from earning her AA degree. They didn't understand that she was a wonderful mother to her preteen daughter. They didn't realize the immense courage it took for her to check into the hospital under an alias because of the threats from the baby's father. They had no idea that she was facing the daunting task of finding a new place to live after the baby was born.

Instead, she was reduced to being just another urban character in a narrative they could easily dismiss. It was disheartening, to say the least, to witness how quickly compassion could slip away in the fast-paced environment of a hospital.

After four more hours of labor, Rochelle was finally completely dilated and effaced. It was time to push. The pushing was intense, and I could see the determination etched on her face. They warned her that the baby would likely be big due to her gestational diabetes, but all she could focus on was the task ahead.

With each push, I encouraged her, reminding her of the strength she had carried with her throughout this journey. Finally, after what felt like an eternity, a beautiful Black baby boy entered the world. He was a big and healthy baby, weighing in at 9 lbs 15 oz. The moment he was placed in Rochelle's arms, pure joy washed over her.

Tears of gratitude rolled down her cheeks as she looked at her miracle, the culmination of her strength, resilience, and love.

In that moment, I was reminded of why we must serve the people in our care with compassion, integrity, and good intentions. It's essential that these values become the standard for all patients, not just those who look like us or fit a specific mold. We need to extend the same level of care and respect to everyone, regardless of their circumstances.

Through this experience, I was able to model advocacy and self-advocacy, showing Rochelle that her voice mattered. I helped her find her strength, the tools she needed to speak up for herself when others failed to recognize her humanity. The treatment she received during her labor and delivery was unacceptable, and it highlighted the disparities that exist in healthcare.

Yet, amidst those challenges, Rochelle emerged victorious. Each time I look at the picture of her precious baby boy, I am reminded of the triumph of his birth—the triumph of a mother who fought against the odds, who refused to be silenced, and who embraced her journey with grace.

This experience served as a powerful reminder that our roles as doulas go beyond support; we must be fierce advocates for our clients. Every woman deserves to be seen, heard, and respected during one of the most significant moments of her life. Together, we can work toward a future where every birth is treated with the dignity it deserves, and where compassion is the norm, not the exception.

CARE TEAM APPROACH AND ASSESSMENT

1. Describe how this Healthcare Center/Birthcare Center/ Hospital responded as a Doula friendly facility.

2. Did the patient experience any barriers to her care?

3. How were any barriers mitigated by the Doula?

4. Describe how the care the mother and family received was positively impacted by the Doula's work.

5. How did the Doula partner with the medical team?

6. How could care have been different for this mom from the Doula or medical team?

7. Describe how she received equitable empathy and respectful care.

CHAPTER 2

A Disrupted Destiny

I met a beautiful and smart young woman named Karen in early 2022. From the moment we connected, I was struck by her gentle spirit and fierce determination. A true go-getter, she was living life on her own terms. Having moved to Los Angeles from the East Coast, Karen was on a mission to start her own business, and everything seemed to be falling into place. She supported herself comfortably and enjoyed the fruits of her labor. She was driving her dream car and living the kind of life that many only aspire to.

Then she met a man. He brought a different kind of energy into her life—one filled with love and care. Though he didn't have much to offer materially, their connection was undeniable. He struggled to make a living for himself, but Karen saw something in him that sparked her affection. His compassion and attention drew her in, and she was captivated by the potential she saw.

As their relationship blossomed, Karen became invested in his success. She took him to job interviews, bought him clothes, and supported him in any way she could. It was an act of love for her, giving without reservation, believing in him even when he struggled to believe in himself.

But then everything changed. Karen discovered she was pregnant, and the news shook their world. Instead of sharing in her joy, he reacted with disbelief and fear. "I don't want a baby," he told her flatly, urging her to have an abortion. He expressed that he didn't want to have anything to do with her, leaving Karen in a state of shock. Just a short while ago, they had seemed so close, so committed to each other—what had happened? Why had he switched up on her so suddenly?

As the days passed, she watched in disbelief as he began to see other women—women who didn't seem to have much going for them. The heartbreak was palpable. Here she was, someone who had given him her all, and he preferred to pursue relationships with those who were less established. It felt like a betrayal, and as he flaunted these new relationships in her face, Karen made the painful decision to end their relationship.

Yet the toll it took on her was immense. In her pursuit of a loving partnership, she had neglected her business, and now it was crumbling around her. The emotional strain, combined with the challenges of impending motherhood, left her feeling utterly lost. She found herself pregnant, without resources, and with nowhere to call home.

In the depths of her despair, Karen's resilience began to shine through. She had always been a fighter, and despite the overwhelming circumstances, she knew she had to take charge of her life again. With every challenge she faced, she grew stronger, determined to rebuild what she had lost.

I often think about Karen and the journey she has been on. She serves as a powerful reminder of how love can sometimes lead us down unexpected paths, and how quickly everything can change. But her story is also one of hope and renewal, a testament to the strength that lies within each of us, waiting to be awakened, even in the darkest of times.

As her doula, I knew my role would be to support her, not just in her pregnancy but in rediscovering her own strength and purpose. Karen's journey would be one of growth, resilience, and ultimately, empowerment. And I was honored to walk alongside her as she navigated this new chapter in her life.

This is where our paths intertwined. I was assigned to work with Karen as her doula, and from our very first meeting, we bonded immediately. There was something about her gentle spirit and unwavering determination that resonated with me. As I got to know her better, she began to share her story, and I could see the pain etched on her face. She felt abandoned, hopeless, and overwhelmed by the weight of her circumstances.

Being in Los Angeles without any family support was a heavy burden to bear. After some time, she decided to go spend time with her family down south, hoping it would help her get back on her feet. However, this meant that she would no longer have access to doula support. I wished her well and encouraged her to stay in touch, hoping to hear from her again.

Two months passed, and to my surprise, I received a message from Karen. She told me that she was back in LA and living in a home for pregnant and parenting women. I felt a rush of relief and joy for her, knowing she had found a supportive environment.

It took a while for us to reconnect. I was in the midst of grieving my mother's death and processing my daughter's recent move down south, which left me feeling a bit lost myself. Finally, we talked, and Karen shared her need for my support during this critical time. We agreed to meet and embark on this journey together.

Karen expressed that she was enjoying her stay at the home. She had developed good relationships with the staff and other women in the program, which provided her a sense of community that she desperately needed. But just three weeks later, everything changed. She began experiencing contractions and was admitted to the hospital, where she was told she was in preterm labor. The news was alarming, and I could feel the anxiety radiating off her as she faced this new challenge.

In the hospital, she was given medication to stop the contractions, and for a week, we waited and hoped for the best. Fortunately, the contractions eventually subsided, allowing her to go home. However, the medication came with its own set of challenges. It caused her painful migraines, which added to her already mounting stress. Throughout the remainder of her pregnancy, she struggled with persistent back pain and debilitating migraines that made each day feel like an uphill battle.

At 40 weeks, she was scheduled for an induction. I arrived at the hospital ready to support her through what I knew would be a significant moment in her life. From the onset, labor was incredibly painful for Karen. She braced herself against the intensity of each contraction, but amidst the pain, she shared her concerns with me.

"Felicia, I have a bump on my vulva," she said, her voice laced with worry. "I feel like something is wrong."

I could see the fear in her eyes as she relayed her concerns to the nurse. It was clear that this was weighing heavily on her mind. In moments like this, it was crucial for me to help advocate for her. I urged the nurse to examine the bump and assess her concerns, ensuring that Karen's voice was heard and her worries addressed.

As the nurses examined her, I held Karen's hand, providing comfort and reassurance. It was moments like these that underscored the importance of having someone by your side who understands your journey. We were in this together, and I would do everything in my power to help her navigate the uncertainties of labor and motherhood.

As the labor continued, I stayed close, reminding her of her strength and the resilience she had shown throughout her journey. Together, we would face whatever challenges lay ahead.

Initially, the nurse downplayed Karen's concern about the bump. They swabbed it and sent the sample to the lab for testing, but I could see the worry etched on her face. When the results came back, they revealed a harsh truth: she tested positive for a very serious sexually transmitted disease. In that moment, my heart sank for her. This news meant she was no longer a candidate for a vaginal delivery; a C-section was now necessary. The weight of it all crushed her. The actions of someone she once cared for had not only affected her heart but had now impacted her health in a profound way.

As she was whisked away to surgery, I felt a deep sense of sorrow for what she was enduring. In the blink of an eye, everything had changed. But amid the devastation, she delivered a gorgeous baby girl, a precious life that emerged from such turmoil.

Doula's Contributions:

After the surgery, I stayed with Karen for a couple of hours, offering her comfort as she began to process everything that had happened. I left the hospital that day, only to reach out later, eager to see how she was doing. It was during this conversation that she learned she had preeclampsia. The news hit her like another blow; she was prescribed magnesium sulfate to treat the condition, and I could hear the frustration and fear in her voice.

She was told that she would be hospitalized until her blood pressure returned to a normal range.

The next three days were spent in an effort to get her preeclampsia under control, but despite their best efforts, it persisted. To make matters worse, the inflammation of her liver began to complicate things further. As if that weren't enough, she received another unsettling piece of news: her baby was going to be released from the hospital, and she needed to arrange for someone to pick her up.

I could hear the despair in her voice. "I don't have anyone here. No family," she said, her words heavy with desperation. It was a harsh reality to confront—being a new mother with a beautiful baby girl, yet feeling utterly alone. A friend agreed to stay overnight to help care for the baby, but Karen knew that this wasn't a long-term solution.

As the days passed, her situation felt increasingly overwhelming. The pressure of having few friends and no family nearby weighed heavily on her. After several sleepless nights and countless tears, she reluctantly reached out to a family member of the baby's father, hoping they would be willing to come and help. It was a decision made from sheer necessity, but it felt like a further blow to her already fragile state.

When the family member finally arrived at the hospital, it was a bittersweet moment. While relief washed over her that help had come, Karen struggled physically and emotionally. The medications made her disoriented, clouding her thoughts, and the inflammation in her liver was a constant reminder of her struggles.

Each time I visited her, I saw the toll that this experience was taking on her. The joyous moment of welcoming her daughter into the world had been overshadowed by an avalanche of complications, fear, and feelings of isolation.

Throughout this ordeal, I remained by her side, advocating for her, reminding her of her strength, and reassuring her that she was not alone.

We navigated the complexities of her care together, and I encouraged her to voice her needs and concerns. She had faced more than her fair share of challenges, but we would face this one together, one day at a time.

On Day 4, everything changed once again. The family member of the baby's dad invited him to come and see the baby—and my client—without her consent. When Karen saw him walk through the door, shock washed over her, quickly followed by a wave of anger and betrayal. She felt utterly blindsided; this was not how she wanted her first interactions as a new mother to go.

As he entered the room, the atmosphere grew heavy with unspoken words. The dad didn't even greet her; he simply stood there, awkwardly silent. The family member attempted to explain their reasoning for inviting him, stating that they thought having him present would make her feel better. But instead, it only heightened her discomfort. In that moment, Karen found her voice. "I'm uncomfortable with you being here," she told them firmly. Turning to the baby's dad, she said, "You need to leave." It was a powerful moment, a reclamation of her space and her feelings.

The emotional toll of that visit was immense, amplifying the physical pain she was already grappling with in the early postpartum period. For the next two weeks, Karen remained in the hospital, battling preeclampsia and liver inflammation.

Each day was a struggle, but finally, after what felt like an eternity, the medication began to take effect, and her health stabilized enough for her to be discharged.

But just as she thought relief was within her grasp, another hurdle appeared. Upon her release, she learned that the maternity home where she had planned to stay was in the middle of a COVID outbreak. Panic surged through her. The thought of being separated from her baby, whom she had fought so hard to bring into the world, felt unbearable.

With nowhere to go, she reached out to a friend who graciously offered her a place to stay until the outbreak subsided. The kindness of that friend was a lifeline during a turbulent time, but the uncertainty continued to weigh heavily on her.

Life had dealt Karen more hardship than anyone should have to bear, yet she pressed on. After nearly three and a half weeks, she finally returned to the maternity home, where she could begin the slow process of recovery.

With each passing day, she grew stronger, not only physically but emotionally as well.

Now a mother to a beautiful baby girl, Karen nurtured her daughter with an unwavering love. Their bond deepened as they shared quiet moments together, filled with laughter and gentle smiles. I felt immense gratitude for being part of her journey to motherhood.

Through her struggles, Karen demonstrated what it meant to be a survivor. She faced her challenges with an incredible grace and strength that inspired everyone around her. It was a privilege to witness her resilience and to support her as she embraced her new role, transforming adversity into empowerment.

CARE TEAM APPROACH AND ASSESSMENT

1. Describe how this Healthcare Center/Birthcare Center/ Hospital responded as a Doula friendly facility.

2. Did the patient experience any barriers to her care?

3. How were any barriers mitigated by the Doula?

4. Describe how the care the mother and family received was positively impacted by the Doula's work.

5. How did the Doula partner with the medical team?

6. How could care have been different for this mom from the Doula or medical team?

7. Describe how she received equitable empathy and respectful care.

CHAPTER 3

Ready for the Catch

In 2019, I embarked on a profound journey by joining one of the first programs in Los Angeles that specifically provided doula support to African American women. It was a groundbreaking initiative, targeting an urgent need within the maternal health system. The maternal mortality and morbidity rates in the United States are disproportionately high for African American women, with African American women being four times more likely to die during labor, delivery, or the postpartum period than women of other races or ethnicities. Indigenous Native American women face similarly grim statistics, coming in as a close second.

I knew the statistics, but seeing these realities firsthand as a community doula was eye-opening. This was my first experience serving in this role, where the focus wasn't only on traditional doula support but also on connecting clients with essential community resources. Community doulas are lifelines, offering far more than just physical and emotional support during pregnancy and childbirth—we connect families to the resources they need to thrive.

As a community doula, my work began with three prenatal visits. Each visit was an opportunity to build a relationship with my clients, offering educational, physical, and emotional support tailored to their unique situations. From teaching about fetal development to discussing nutrition and the importance of exercise during pregnancy, we covered it all. For many women, this was their first introduction to some of these topics. The effects of adverse substances during pregnancy, warning signs for preterm labor and delivery, and essential infant care skills were also key components of our conversations.

But education wasn't where it ended. As doulas, we were also present for one of the most critical moments in our clients' lives: labor and delivery.

The continuous care we provided during that time allowed us to advocate for our clients in real-time, ensuring their voices were heard in spaces that often overlooked them. Advocacy was central to our role, and I quickly learned that it wasn't just about empowering the women—it was about modeling self-advocacy so they could continue to advocate for themselves long after we were no longer in the picture.

Postpartum care was just as essential. During the three postpartum visits, we focused on topics that many new mothers found overwhelming: newborn care, breastfeeding, and understanding postpartum depression. We addressed the physical recovery of the mother, a subject often under-discussed in mainstream healthcare. Many women were surprised to learn about the wide range of normal postpartum experiences, from the physical pain to the emotional rollercoasters.

For me, each visit wasn't just about providing information; it was about making sure my clients felt heard and supported. By connecting them with community-based organizations and additional resources, we helped bridge gaps in healthcare and foster a support network that many of them lacked.

The stories and struggles I encountered were as diverse as the women I served, but the common thread was resilience. These women, despite facing systemic barriers and personal hardships, were committed to providing a better future for their children. Being able to stand with them during such a pivotal moment in their lives was nothing short of humbling.

Looking back, this program and my role in it reshaped my understanding of what it means to care for a community. It wasn't just about the births, the babies, or even the health statistics. It was about creating a circle of care that acknowledged and supported the whole woman—her mind, body, spirit, and circumstances.

This work—this sacred calling—goes beyond statistics. It's about rewriting the narrative for African American women and their babies. It's about ensuring that each woman feels valued, heard, and empowered. That, above all, was and continues to be the heart of community doula work.

As I sat with Bridgette, one of the first things she said was how afraid she was of giving birth, particularly because of all the news and talk surrounding mortality and morbidity rates among African American women. It was a fear I had heard many times before, but it still struck me deeply each time. Our program was created precisely to address and offset this trend. Research shows that when African American women receive support from African American doulas, birth outcomes improve significantly. This program was, in a way, a lifeline for women like Bridgette, providing not just care but hope.

The program is available to all African American women, regardless of socioeconomic or educational background, and Bridgette was a perfect candidate. She'd faced a lot of hardship, losing her mother at a young age and spending much of her childhood in foster care. Her past had instilled in her a deep commitment to her children's well-being, ensuring they had the stability and care she didn't always receive growing up.

In addition to being a dedicated mother, she was also in college, taking online courses to eventually work with families. She wanted to be a pillar of support for others, just as she was striving to be for her children.

Then came the call that she thought she was in labor.

I decided to join her immediately. When I arrived, her contractions were about every 10 minutes, each lasting around 30 seconds. It seemed like the early stages, so we settled in, spending the next few hours talking, eating, and using comfort measures like breathing techniques to help her navigate through each contraction.

As we passed the time, her children returned home from school. Bridgette proudly introduced me to her four lively children—bright, funny, and full of energy. Their presence seemed to lift her spirits, providing a welcome distraction from the intensifying labor. She was able to focus on their antics and laughter, which helped ease some of the tension and nerves. But even as we all laughed together, I could tell her contractions were becoming more intense and frequent.

We talked through it, using deep breaths and positions to help manage the growing discomfort. I was glad I was there to provide the calm, continuous support she needed as her labor progressed. We were entering the next phase, where everything becomes more focused and deliberate.

This particular client lived with her partner, and they were going through a challenging time in their relationship. His daughter from a previous relationship had moved in with them, and the dynamics in the home had shifted dramatically. The children were aged between 3 and 12, and his daughter's behavior was causing issues—particularly her tendency to lie and accuse the other children of hurting her. It created a lot of conflict, and my client was caught in the middle, trying to protect her children while also encouraging her partner to seek help for his daughter. Unfortunately, he downplayed the situation, which only added more tension to their home life.

The day her labor truly began, I arrived to find her experiencing contractions, though they were still relatively spaced out. She told me she needed to use the bathroom, and after being in there for 30 minutes, she came out looking different. Her body had progressed—her mucus plug had come out, and her contractions were much stronger.

I encouraged her to go to the hospital, and I let her partner know as well. Together, we gathered her things, and I had her partner load them into the car.

As we got to the car, she stood there, clearly uncomfortable, saying she couldn't sit down. For about 20 minutes, we tried to get her to sit, but the contractions were becoming so intense that she could barely speak. I knew it was time to get her to the hospital, but as soon as she got into the car, she suddenly said something was wrong. When I looked, I could see the baby's head emerging.

In that moment, everything slowed down, and I realized I had to make a quick decision. If I didn't act, the baby would fall onto the floor of the car. There was no time to second-guess. I told her partner to call 911, and then I instinctively moved into action. As she pushed, I caught the baby—gently grabbing it around the waist and pulling it out, then placing the baby on my client's chest. I couldn't believe what had just happened.

Within five minutes of her sitting in the car, the baby had been born. I wrapped the baby in a towel as we waited for the ambulance to arrive, which felt like the longest 10 minutes. When the paramedics arrived, they checked both my client and the baby, and although everything seemed fine, they took her to the hospital for a more thorough examination. On the way to the hospital, she delivered the placenta in the ambulance.

Though my client initially wanted to be taken to MLK Community Hospital, the paramedics had to bring her to Centinela Hospital, as it was closer. She was upset at first but eventually agreed that it was the safest decision. I followed the ambulance to the hospital, and when I arrived, I was relieved to hear that both my client and her baby girl were in perfect health after a full examination.

In the midst of this whirlwind, I couldn't believe I had just caught a baby. I had also cut the umbilical cord and held this beautiful little girl in my arms—it felt so surreal. Her partner was there, but understandably shocked by how quickly everything unfolded.

I've always been able to remain calm during unexpected situations, and in this moment, it was as though I went into autopilot mode—free from fear or anxiety.

It was only after the birth, when we were at the hospital, that I truly processed what had happened. My client even jokingly mentioned that I should become the baby's 'TiTi,' an honorary aunt, a role I embraced with joy.

The following day, I returned to the hospital to sign the birth certificate as a witness to the birth. It was truly a once-in-a-lifetime event, and I felt blessed to have been there to help bring that beautiful baby girl into the world. Fast forward five years, and that same baby just finished her first year of kindergarten.

In 2022, I had the honor of supporting my client again when she delivered her sixth child. The bond between a doula and her client is something special—it's a partnership based on trust, and I am grateful to have been a part of her journey, not once but twice.

CARE TEAM APPROACH AND ASSESSMENT

1. Describe how this Healthcare Center/Birthcare Center/ Hospital responded as a Doula friendly facility.

2. Did the patient experience any barriers to her care?

3. How were any barriers mitigated by the Doula?

4. Describe how the care the mother and family received was positively impacted by the Doula's work.

5. How did the Doula partner with the medical team?

6. How could care have been different for this mom from the Doula or medical team?

7. Describe how she received equitable empathy and respectful care.

CHAPTER 4

Relationships are Everything

Dynamics in relationships can greatly affect a pregnancy, sometimes in ways that aren't immediately apparent. When I first met Zoe, the tension between her and her partner was unmistakable. She wanted more commitment—a marriage, not to be a single mom. But her partner wasn't ready for that level of commitment yet, feeling it was too soon in their relationship to even consider marriage. As a compromise, they decided to live together, which brought its own set of challenges.

Throughout her pregnancy, Zoe faced constant discomfort, both physically and emotionally. She felt that her partner lacked compassion and didn't recognize how much her pregnancy had changed her. He seemed to expect her to continue doing things as she had before the pregnancy, without any real consideration of how her growing body and the toll of pregnancy were affecting her. This became a significant point of contention, as Zoe also felt like her partner wasn't doing much to make their home more comfortable for her. Instead of preparing a nurturing environment, she felt like he was taking her for granted—spending too much time with his friends and focusing more on his business than on her or the baby.

The tensions between them escalated, with frequent arguments centered on their differing expectations. Zoe was frustrated not only with his lack of emotional support but also with their starkly different approaches to keeping their home. She valued order and cleanliness, while he was more laid-back, content to let things slide. This divide grew deeper after a pipe burst, causing their home to flood. As they were forced to relocate temporarily while repairs were made, the added stress seemed to push them further apart.

During this already turbulent time, we received a unique opportunity. We were invited to be featured on a national television show, which focused on highlighting the challenges African American women face during pregnancy, especially around mortality and morbidity. It was an amazing platform to bring awareness to the issues affecting Black women during childbirth, and it gave us both a chance to talk openly about our experiences.

The exposure allowed Zoe to not only share her personal story but to also put a face to the statistics that so many African American women face. But amidst the excitement, Zoe's health took a turn.

At 26 weeks, she began experiencing intense contractions. Worried, she went to see her doctor, only to be told that her cervix was shortening—a potential sign that she could go into preterm labor. She was admitted to the hospital and treated.

Thankfully, after some time, the contractions stopped, and she was released, but the scare of possibly having her baby early left her and her partner overwhelmed and anxious.

The next few weeks, however, saw a strange twist. When Zoe went for a follow-up appointment, her doctor informed her that her cervix hadn't shortened after all. The conflicting information left her frustrated, as she felt like she'd been through unnecessary stress. While the health scare subsided, the tension in her relationship did not.

By 30 weeks, things between Zoe and her partner had reached a boiling point. Feeling more unsure about their future than ever, she gave him an ultimatum—either they get married now, or she was prepared to end the relationship. This demand made an already tense situation worse. Seeking emotional support, Zoe reached out to her family, as well as her partner's parents. She hoped that they might help mediate, or at least provide some guidance as she navigated this difficult chapter in her life.

It was clear that, for Zoe, her relationship struggles were as consuming as her pregnancy. While her body prepared for the arrival of her child, her heart and mind were caught up in whether or not she and her partner could find a way forward together. Pregnancy is challenging enough, but when you add relationship difficulties, it can magnify every emotion.

In Zoe's case, the uncertainty about her future with her partner weighed heavily on her, making the entire experience that much more complex.

One of the barriers for Zoe's partner was rooted in his own past. He didn't find out who his father was until he was an adult, and this left him with unresolved feelings about becoming a father, particularly since they were having a son. Zoe tried multiple times to talk to him about this, but he simply refused to engage in the conversation. It left her feeling confused and isolated in the relationship, as their connection seemed to ebb and flow with no real consistency.

Over the next 10 weeks, Zoe and I spent a lot of time talking about their relationship dynamics. I encouraged them to seek counseling, and eventually, they did find a therapist.

The sessions brought a lot of underlying issues to the surface. Communication was a major hurdle for both of them. Zoe's partner admitted that he didn't respond well to ultimatums, while Zoe felt her concerns were being dismissed. Despite their efforts, they eventually reached an impasse. They were unable to find a way to accommodate each other's needs and, as a result, decided to step away from therapy.

When Zoe went into labor at 40 weeks, it initially seemed like things were progressing quickly.

We all thought the birth would happen soon, but about five hours into labor, the baby began experiencing decelerations—its heart rate would drop during contractions. Normally, the baby's heart rate should have been around 130 beats per minute (bpm), but it would drop to 90 bpm with each contraction.

As labor continued, the decelerations became more frequent, and it took longer for the baby's heart rate to recover between contractions. Zoe's labor stalled at 7 cm, and after several hours without any progress, I began to discuss the possibility of needing a C-section. This news brought her partner to tears. Despite all the previous tension, his compassion and empathy in that moment were palpable. It was one of those rare bonding moments where everything else fell away, and they were able to connect.

They reached out to Zoe's family and asked for prayers. Amazingly, her labor picked up again, and within an hour, she was fully dilated and ready to deliver. However, the baby's heart rate continued to decelerate, so the doctor decided to use vacuum suction to assist with the delivery. Fortunately, Zoe gathered the strength to push, and with the help of the suction, she was able to deliver the baby.

Their son was born with respiratory problems, and the NICU team had to step in right away. For the first hour, they monitored him closely, and thankfully, his breathing improved. Zoe was finally able to have skin-to-skin contact with him, which was a beautiful moment of relief.

They spent the first two hours alone with their newborn—part of the hospital's baby-friendly protocol, designed to allow parents and babies to bond through skin-to-skin and eye contact. It was a precious time for them as a new family, and I could see that it helped Zoe's partner connect in ways he hadn't been able to during the pregnancy.

Zoe was discharged from the hospital after two days, and a week later, the repairs on their home were finally complete, allowing them to move back in. Throughout the postpartum period, I stayed in touch, visiting them regularly. Each time, we used a screening tool to assess for signs of postpartum baby blues or depression, and thankfully, Zoe consistently tested negative. She physically recovered quickly and was almost back to her pre-pregnancy activity level in no time.

Unfortunately, despite the beautiful moments they shared during the birth, Zoe and her partner couldn't resolve their differences.

They eventually went their separate ways. As doulas, we often provide emotional support, but sometimes the issues in a relationship go beyond what we can help with. In those cases, I always encourage my clients to seek professional mental health support. Sadly, in this case, the unresolved problems caused an irreparable breakdown in their relationship.

Now, they're learning how to navigate co-parenting one day at a time. It's not easy, but they are committed to making it work for the sake of their son. Zoe is resilient, and I know she'll continue to face each challenge with the same grace she's shown throughout her journey.

CARE TEAM APPROACH AND ASSESSMENT

1. Describe how this Healthcare Center/Birthcare Center/ Hospital responded as a Doula friendly facility.

2. Did the patient experience any barriers to her care?

3. How were any barriers mitigated by the Doula?

4. Describe how the care the mother and family received was positively impacted by the Doula's work.

5. How did the Doula partner with the medical team?

6. How could care have been different for this mom from the Doula or medical team?

7. Describe how she received equitable empathy and respectful care.

CHAPTER 5

Sacrifices

When I first met my client, Victoria, she was five months pregnant and unhoused. She had recently been admitted into a maternity home, which provided her with some much-needed support. Victoria had been in a relationship with the baby's father, but they weren't able to resolve their differences.

When the relationship ended, he cut off all communication with her and essentially abandoned her. She was left with no place to live, and the emotional toll was immense. Thankfully, she managed to get into the maternity home where she could receive shelter and care.

Victoria's heartbreak ran deep. She had spent much of her childhood and teenage years in foster care, as her mother struggled with mental health issues and was unable to care for her children. Victoria's time in foster care shaped her personality in profound ways, making it difficult for her to trust others. She had become fiercely self-reliant, which made it hard for her to accept the support I offered as her doula.

Our doula-client relationship didn't get off to the best start. I would reach out to her, but she wouldn't return my calls. Eventually, I managed to connect with her and explain more about our doula program. Once she understood what the program entailed, she warmed up to the idea and became more open to receiving support. As doulas, we wear many hats—we're advocates, educators, encouragers, and, most importantly, a consistent support system. I wanted Victoria to know that I was here for her, no matter what.

Like many of my clients, Victoria had a strained relationship with her mother. She didn't receive any guidance or support from her, which left her feeling uninformed and isolated. When she found out she was pregnant, she felt conflicted. She had always wanted a family structure, and being a single mom wasn't part of the plan. Family meant a lot to her, and she longed for stability and support.

This is where her godmother came in. At one point in Victoria's life, she had lived with her godmother as a foster child, and they had maintained a close relationship. Her godmother was invested in her well-being and stepped in to help when Victoria needed it most. She provided a stable home, offering her a spacious two-bedroom house to live in. Victoria was excited about this prospect—getting back on her feet and regaining her independence. However, she was also anxious about doing everything on her own. The idea of being solely responsible for her baby was daunting, but her desire for independence gave her the motivation to push forward.

We met regularly for our prenatal visits, and each time we spent a significant amount of time preparing for labor and delivery, breastfeeding, and the postpartum period. Since I was going to be her only support person during labor, I wanted to make sure she felt equipped and confident going into the birth. We discussed comfort measures, breathing techniques, and what to expect at each stage of labor.

Despite her challenges and initial hesitation, Victoria was determined to make the best of her situation. I could see her strength, even though she had moments of vulnerability. By the end of our visits, she seemed more empowered and ready to face the journey ahead.

During one of our prenatal visits, Victoria shared her concerns about pain management. She had undergone back surgery years before and was worried that she wouldn't be able to get an epidural. This led us to dedicate a lot of time to going over comfort measures and various breathing techniques. I encouraged her to practice these techniques, knowing they might make a difference when the time came.

At 39 weeks, her doctor scheduled an induction, which can involve various methods, both natural and medical, to help start labor. Induction can be more painful than natural labor, especially when Pitocin is involved. Pitocin, a synthetic version of oxytocin, causes contractions to be more intense. For someone without pain management options, the experience can be excruciating.

When Victoria was admitted to the hospital, she wasn't dilated or effaced, meaning her cervix hadn't yet started to open or thin. The medical team began with Cytotec to help soften the cervix. Victoria was able to manage this stage without too much discomfort, but once they used the Foley catheter, or the 'balloon method,' to further dilate her cervix, her contractions began in earnest. By the time she was 3 cm dilated, the pain was significant, and she was given Pitocin to help things along.

As the intensity of the contractions increased, Victoria's discomfort became unbearable. She began to cry and asked for pain relief. First, she was given Nitrous Oxide, which provided some initial relief by taking the edge off her pain. But after a few hours, and at 6 cm dilated, it was no longer effective.

Her doctor then ordered IV narcotics—Morphine—providing temporary relief and allowing her to get some rest between contractions. However, as her labor progressed, the Morphine wore off, and her pain levels skyrocketed again. We tried everything—massage, aromatherapy, movement—but nothing helped. At this point, she was in so much pain she was lying on the floor, crying hysterically.

Her nurse didn't seem to know how to handle her intense reaction and, at one point, appeared to be frustrated with her. Victoria sensed the nurse's irritation and confided in me, feeling that her pain wasn't being taken seriously. I asked Victoria if she wanted to address it herself or have me advocate for her. When the nurse came back in, I explained how Victoria felt. To her credit, the nurse immediately apologized and assured Victoria that she didn't mean to come across that way. From then on, the nurse became one of Victoria's biggest supporters.

As the pain escalated, the doctor called an anesthesiologist to evaluate whether Victoria could get an epidural despite her previous back surgery.

Thankfully, she was cleared for the epidural, and after 48 hours of agonizing labor, she was finally able to find relief. Just two hours after receiving the epidural, Victoria delivered a beautiful and healthy baby girl.

Victoria's birth was one of the hardest I've ever experienced as a doula. If it was that challenging with me there, I can't imagine how she would have coped on her own.

During our first postpartum visit, we discussed her labor. She expressed how the pain had made her feel completely out of control and described it as the hardest thing she had ever endured. She thanked me for being there, and I assured her that despite everything, she had handled it with strength and resilience. I reminded her of how courageous she had been throughout the entire experience.

In moments like this, when labor is especially difficult, the support of a doula can be transformative. No one should have to go through something like that alone. That's why it's so important for doula services to be available to anyone who seeks them. With the right support, even the most challenging labors can be navigated with greater ease and confidence.

CARE TEAM APPROACH AND ASSESSMENT

1. Describe how this Healthcare Center/Birthcare Center/ Hospital responded as a Doula friendly facility.

2. Did the patient experience any barriers to her care?

3. How were any barriers mitigated by the Doula?

4. Describe how the care the mother and family received was positively impacted by the Doula's work.

5. How did the Doula partner with the medical team?

6. How could care have been different for this mom from the Doula or medical team?

7. Describe how she received equitable empathy and respectful care.

CHAPTER 6

Safe Hands

I first met Wynette when she was twelve weeks pregnant. From the moment we began talking, it was clear that she carried a deep emotional burden alongside her pregnancy. Wynette shared that she was living with her family, but her relationship with her mother was strained. Her mother suffered from anxiety, isolating herself and rarely leaving the house unless it was absolutely necessary. Wynette said that growing up, her mother wasn't there for her or her siblings the way they needed. The mental illness had created a moody and distant atmosphere in their home, making communication almost impossible.

Wynette described how painful it was living there. Her mother's inability to be emotionally present had left scars, especially during her formative years. On top of her mother's mental health struggles, Wynette had endured physical and sexual abuse. She explained how those traumas had devastated her, and she carried a lot of resentment toward her mother for not being able to protect her. Despite these experiences, Wynette was determined to be a better mother to her own child.

At forty years old, Wynette looked incredibly youthful, and I initially thought she was in her twenties. She was self-employed, running a production company, but finances were often uncertain. Some months were great, while others barely brought in enough money to cover basic needs. This led to frequent arguments between her and her mother, adding even more tension to their already fragile relationship.

One of the first things Wynette told me was that she wanted to be well-prepared for the birth of her baby. She was open to learning all she could about pregnancy, breastfeeding, and infant care. We spent a lot of time discussing these topics, and I could see how determined she was to provide a stable, loving environment for her child—something she hadn't experienced growing up.

Wynette was in a relationship with a younger man, and although their relationship had started beautifully, things began to change after she disclosed her pregnancy. He felt unprepared to be a father and wanted to wait until they were in a better financial situation. Although Wynette hoped they could work things out, she noticed they were beginning to drift apart. He was supportive in some ways, but as the pregnancy progressed, he withdrew. He never attended any of our prenatal sessions, even though she invited him every time.

Despite his emotional distance, Wynette remained focused. She decided that whether her partner would be involved or not, she would be fully prepared for labor and parenting on her own. She enrolled in classes at Black Infant Health (BIH), an incredible resource for Black mothers that provides education and support along with essential items like diapers and baby clothes. At her age, she was considered high-risk, so she underwent genetic testing and was relieved to find out she was having a healthy baby girl. However, her specialist raised concerns about the baby's size, suggesting that her placenta might not be providing enough nutrients.

At 38 weeks, Wynette's OB/GYN recommended inducing labor, but Wynette was firm in her belief that she should carry her baby to full term. Her doctor also told her she would need to deliver at a hospital in East LA, which didn't have a NICU or the resources to handle high-risk pregnancies. Wynette, however, had done her research and decided that she wanted to deliver at Long Beach Memorial, which was better equipped. Her OB/GYN didn't deliver there, so she'd have to show up in active labor with her medical records in hand.

Determined, Wynette moved in with a friend in Long Beach when she reached 39 weeks to be closer to the hospital. She even tried a natural method to induce labor, drinking a midwife's brew made of castor oil, lemon verbena oil, almond butter, and apricot juice. Initially, nothing happened, but after two hours, her contractions began, coming every five minutes and lasting a minute each. I instructed her to go to the hospital immediately. When she arrived, she was dilated 6 cm and 70% effaced, with the baby still high at -2. She was officially in active labor.

For the first couple of hours, everything seemed to be progressing smoothly. But in the third hour, the baby's heart rate began to decelerate dangerously during contractions, and it was taking a long time for the baby to recover between them. The medical staff closely monitored her for two more hours as these deep decelerations continued. Wynette's OB/GYN was committed to honoring her desire for a vaginal birth, but the baby's safety became the top concern when the heart rate dropped into the 70s and stayed low for too long.

The doctor recommended a C-section, and though Wynette was initially disappointed, she knew it was the best decision for her baby. By this time, her baby's father had finally arrived at the hospital, although he chose not to go into the operating room with her. As they prepped her for surgery, I was allowed to stay by her side.

The baby was delivered within ten minutes, but the room was eerily silent. I could see the baby from where I sat—she wasn't crying, wasn't breathing, and her tiny body was limp. The medical team worked on her for ten long minutes, trying to resuscitate her, but there was no response. The NICU team rushed in, took over, and quickly moved the baby to the NICU for further treatment. Wynette was devastated, and I reassured her that I would go to the NICU to check on her baby while she recovered from surgery.

When I got to the NICU, I learned that the baby would be staying there for several days. Given her lack of oxygen at birth, there was concern that there might be brain damage, and the hospital followed a protocol of lowering the baby's body temperature to mitigate potential brain injury.

When I returned to Wynette, she was understandably anxious about her baby being alone, but it was too early for her to be able to go see her.

At that point, the baby's father returned. Wynette asked him to go check on the baby, but he shockingly responded that he needed to leave for New York to close a deal. Wynette was furious. He downplayed the baby's condition, minimizing Wynette's concerns. He stayed with the baby for only 45 minutes before leaving the hospital.

Wynette was heartbroken, but she remained strong for her daughter. I spent the next few hours comforting her. The next day, she was able to see her baby, who was stable and not showing any signs of brain damage. Thankfully, both Wynette and her daughter were going to be okay.

This birth was hard. It was a reminder of how vulnerable birthing individuals are, and how vital it is to have a strong support system. Wynette's determination, strength, and trust in her own instincts carried her through, and I was grateful she allowed me to be part of her journey.

CARE TEAM APPROACH AND ASSESSMENT

1. Describe how this Healthcare Center/Birthcare Center/ Hospital responded as a Doula friendly facility.

2. Did the patient experience any barriers to her care?

3. How were any barriers mitigated by the Doula?

4. Describe how the care the mother and family received was positively impacted by the Doula's work.

5. How did the Doula partner with the medical team?

6. How could care have been different for this mom from the Doula or medical team?

7. Describe how she received equitable empathy and respectful care.

CHAPTER 7

Anxious Deliveries

I met Gina when she was 20 weeks pregnant, and from our very first meeting, I could sense that anxiety had a firm hold on her. It wasn't uncommon in the aftermath of COVID-19, especially for pregnant women, who often found themselves overwhelmed with worry about their health and their unborn child. Gina, like many other African American women, was acutely aware of the statistics. The media coverage about Black maternal mortality weighed heavily on her, and the fear of becoming one of those statistics consumed her.

From the outset, Gina spoke about her overwhelming thoughts, the stories she had read, and the disparities in birth outcomes for African American women. She feared dying during childbirth, a fear that was unfortunately not unfounded given the systemic racism and biases that exist in gynecology and obstetrics. I knew from the start that my role with Gina would be to help her manage this fear, to arm her with knowledge, and to build her confidence.

We bonded instantly, and she introduced me to her partner, George. I started affectionately calling them "GG" — Gina and George. They were a delightful couple, eager to learn and open to my support. But it was clear that Gina's anxiety, rooted in very real concerns, would require special attention. She had been consuming so much media about maternal deaths, and I wanted to offer her reassurance.

I shared with Gina the painful history of how racism in healthcare has shaped the present-day disparities we see. I told her about Dr. J. Marion Sims, who is often called the father of modern gynecology. He performed surgical experiments on enslaved Black women without anesthesia because he believed that Black women didn't feel pain like white women. This belief still permeates the healthcare system today, as studies have shown that Black patients are often undertreated for pain. When Black women in labor cry out, they are often ignored. Gina was shocked but appreciative of the education, and it seemed to ease some of her fears.

As we continued working together, I emphasized that the problem wasn't her Black body; it was the racism embedded in the medical system. I explained how today's biases manifest — in doctors not listening to their Black patients, in dismissing their concerns, and in delaying life-saving interventions. I even told her about the 2023 case of April Valentine, a young Black woman in Los Angeles who lost her life due to medical negligence during labor. Despite doing everything right, April's cries for help were ignored, and she tragically died after a preventable medical emergency. Gina winced when she heard this story and said, "Please, Felicia, make sure that doesn't happen to me." Her eyes pleaded with me, and I vowed to be her advocate.

At our second meeting, I met George again, but this time both their families were present. Some of the women in her family were skeptical about her decision to use a doula, so I invited them to join our session to help ease their concerns. At first, there was visible reluctance, but as we delved into labor and delivery techniques, relaxation exercises, and breathing methods, their skepticism melted away. By the end of the session, we were all sharing birth stories, and I could see the trust forming. It was a beautiful moment of unity, and I could tell that it strengthened Gina's resolve.

As Gina's due date approached, she became more confident in her ability to handle labor and delivery. On the morning of September 25th, she called me at 2:30 AM. "I think I'm in labor," she said, her voice trembling slightly. I talked her through her symptoms, and it was clear she was. Despite my urging, she was hesitant to go to the hospital. Luckily, George was able to convince her, and they went straight to triage. She was 5 centimeters dilated when they arrived, and she was handling her contractions like a pro, determined to have a medication-free labor.

Things became intense when Gina started experiencing back labor. The doctor confirmed that the baby was in an occipital posterior position — face up — which can make contractions more painful. Without any medication, the doctor successfully rotated the baby, and Gina, with incredible strength, tolerated the procedure. I was so proud of her. Her contractions grew more painful, but with George by her side, coaching her through each one, they were a dynamic team. After 17 hours of labor, she delivered a strong, healthy baby girl. It was an awe-inspiring moment.

During one of our postpartum visits, Gina reflected on how she had managed to navigate the anxiety that had once seemed so overwhelming. She admitted that she had moments of doubt, but with the support of George and her family, she found strength she didn't know she had. Her labor was hard, but she did it with peace and grace. I couldn't have been prouder.

Their daughter is a beautiful testament to Black love and resilience. Gina and George are two of the best parents I know, and I can already see how they will thrive as a family. The gratitude they expressed to me, and the love and appreciation from their family, warmed my heart. It reminded me why I do this work. I was honored to be part of their journey, and I will always remember the strength and grace Gina showed as she brought new life into the world.

CARE TEAM APPROACH AND ASSESSMENT

1. Describe how this Healthcare Center/Birthcare Center/ Hospital responded as a Doula friendly facility.

2. Did the patient experience any barriers to her care?

3. How were any barriers mitigated by the Doula?

4. Describe how the care the mother and family received was positively impacted by the Doula's work.

5. How did the Doula partner with the medical team?

6. How could care have been different for this mom from the Doula or medical team?

7. Describe how she received equitable empathy and respectful care.

CHAPTER 8

Complex Conditions

My client Traci was assigned to me during the end of her first trimester, and from the beginning, her pregnancy was complex. She had a health condition that left her with a pain pump in her lower spine, regularly administering medication. This made her pregnancy high-risk and required special medical attention.

During our first call, Traci explained that because of her condition, she faced the difficult decision of either delivering unmedicated or undergoing a C-section, as an epidural was not an option due to her pain pump. Her situation arose after a severe allergic reaction to medication that left her in chronic pain, even unable to walk for a time. Months of physical therapy helped her regain her mobility, but the pain pump remained, and it complicated her pregnancy.

Her doctors — a general OB/GYN and a high-risk OB/GYN — kept insisting that she needed a C-section, particularly her primary OB, who seemed dismissive of her wishes. He constantly pressured her to schedule the surgery, warning that without the epidural, her pain would be unbearable if she tried to labor naturally. Traci felt unheard and frustrated by his approach. He treated her like a child, even though she was 28, simply because she looked younger. It was a demeaning experience for her.

We talked about how doctors sometimes dismiss their patients' feelings, especially Black women, and how important it was for her to advocate for herself. I encouraged her to take her mother or me to her next appointment. At that appointment, with her mother present, the doctor's demeanor completely changed. He listened for the first time, dropping the incessant talk of a C-section. Traci's confidence grew from this experience, and we spent our prenatal appointments focusing on self-advocacy and reaffirming her right to be heard.

Traci's pregnancy came as a surprise. She had been in a long-term relationship for five years without conceiving, so she assumed she couldn't get pregnant. But after casually dating the baby's father, she found herself unexpectedly pregnant. Their relationship was strained from the beginning. Their personalities clashed — she was optimistic, a "cup half full" kind of person, while he tended to be more negative, which led to frequent arguments. He often felt left out, but he resisted getting involved with her family. They also disagreed about parenting, causing further tension between them.

As Traci approached labor, her concern shifted to the induction her doctor had scheduled. She feared the pain would be unbearable, even with all the breathing and relaxation techniques we had practiced. Still, she remained hopeful, determined to give her best effort.

At 38 weeks, Traci was admitted to the hospital, and the induction began with Cytotec to soften her cervix. They then used a balloon catheter to get her to 3 centimeters, followed by Pitocin to start contractions. For a while, everything went smoothly. She handled the contractions well, using movement, positioning, and her breathing techniques. But after three hours, the pain intensified beyond what she could tolerate.

When she was checked, she was 7 centimeters dilated, 60% effaced, and the baby was still high at -2 station. Overwhelmed by the pain, Traci started to cry, feeling like she had let everyone down because she couldn't continue laboring without pain relief. We reassured her that she had done an incredible job — getting to 7 centimeters without an epidural was a huge achievement. She had given it her all.

Ultimately, Traci was prepped for a C-section. Because she couldn't receive an epidural or spinal block due to her pain pump, she had to undergo the surgery under general anesthesia. The surgery took longer than expected, but when she awoke, groggy but alert, she finally got to hold her son. The joy on her face as she did skin-to-skin contact with him was priceless. Both she and the baby's father were ecstatic, holding their healthy son and reveling in the moment.

Despite the challenges and her initial fears, Traci felt at peace with the outcome. She had labored courageously and given it her best, and now she had a healthy baby boy. I reminded her of her strength, and we all celebrated the fact that she had endured an induction without an epidural, making it to 7 centimeters before needing the surgery. Traci had shown tremendous patience and grace throughout the process, and in the end, her reward was the beautiful life of her son.

Afterward, she whispered to me, "I couldn't have done this without you. Thank you so much." Her words humbled me and filled me with gratitude. Supporting her through this journey was an honor, and I was deeply thankful for the positive outcome for her and her family.

CARE TEAM APPROACH AND ASSESSMENT

1. Describe how this Healthcare Center/Birthcare Center/ Hospital responded as a Doula friendly facility.

2. Did the patient experience any barriers to her care?

3. How were any barriers mitigated by the Doula?

4. Describe how the care the mother and family received was positively impacted by the Doula's work.

5. How did the Doula partner with the medical team?

6. How could care have been different for this mom from the Doula or medical team?

7. Describe how she received equitable empathy and respectful care.

CHAPTER 9

The COVID Challenge

Being a doula during the COVID-19 pandemic brought unique challenges, and for much of 2020 and 2021, we had to support our clients virtually. It was a tough transition since we were used to being physically present during labor and delivery. Hospital restrictions were inconsistent, with frequent changes in policy about allowing partners or doulas to attend births. This added confusion and frustration, especially for clients who were already anxious about their deliveries. Despite the difficulties, we made it work, offering virtual support and equipping our clients to advocate for themselves if we couldn't be there.

One couple I'll never forget during that time was Stephan and Erica. Erica had hyperemesis gravidarum, a condition that caused severe nausea and vomiting during pregnancy, making it hard for her to keep food down. For the first trimester, she was so sick that Stephan had to take care of her—bathing her, washing her hair, and feeding her. It was a difficult time for both of them, especially since they didn't know much about pregnancy, labor, or breastfeeding.

We began working together when she entered her second trimester, and her condition had started to improve. Erica's energy began to return, and we started having our prenatal visits virtually, focusing on labor, delivery, breastfeeding, and postpartum care. It was initially challenging to provide support online, but Stephan and Erica were so eager to learn that we spent hours covering everything they needed to know. My main concern was preparing them in case Erica had to labor and deliver without support from her partner or me, given the fluctuating hospital rules.

Despite the inconsistent policies around doulas in hospitals, we managed to prepare them thoroughly, with a strong focus on comfort measures and self-advocacy. We practiced breathing techniques, labor positions, and strategies for managing contractions. Though it was harder to demonstrate virtually, we worked through it, and their confidence grew.

When Erica reached the final weeks of her pregnancy, I was on call 24/7. At 4:30 a.m. one morning, Erica called to say her contractions had intensified, and they were now lasting longer and coming closer together. I instructed her to go to the hospital, and fortunately, the policy allowed both Stephan and me to be present.

When I arrived, Erica was in active labor, dilated to 6 cm, and 80% effaced. She was deeply focused on her contractions and didn't want anyone talking to her. I gently reminded her about the breathing and comfort techniques we had practiced. After some convincing, she was able to get on top of the contractions, which were coming fast and hard.

At one point, Stephan tried to comfort her by rubbing her leg, and Erica yelled at him to stop touching her. The intensity of the moment had her shouting at the nurses as well. But the staff understood, and when the nurse checked her again, Erica was fully dilated—10 cm and 100% effaced. It was time to push.

I held one leg, the nurse held the other, and Stephan stood beside her, offering encouragement. Erica pushed with determination, and soon, the baby began to crown. When she experienced the "ring of fire"—the intense burning sensation as the baby's head emerged—she cried out and stopped pushing. I reminded her about the sensation and encouraged her to keep going. After just three more pushes, her baby boy was born.

The room filled with joy as Stephan and Erica looked at their son for the first time. Erica hadn't torn, and the baby was healthy. They placed him on her chest, and Stephan and Erica both cried with happiness. Despite the strain of labor, Erica turned to the nurse, introduced herself, and apologized for yelling earlier. Everyone laughed, understanding the stress and intensity of childbirth.

In that moment, all the challenges Erica had faced—her hyperemesis gravidarum, the stress of pregnancy during COVID, and the unpredictability of hospital policies—faded away. She now had her reward, her beautiful baby boy, and their family felt complete. It was a privilege to be a part of their journey, and their gratitude was humbling. Despite everything, love and resilience shone through, reminding me why I do this work.

CARE TEAM APPROACH AND ASSESSMENT

1. Describe how this Healthcare Center/BirthCare Center/Hospital responded as a Doula friendly facility.

2. Did the patient experience any barriers to her care?

3. How was this mitigated by the Doula?

4. Describe how the care the mother and family received was positively impacted by the Doula's work.

5. How did the Doula partner with the medical team?

6. How could care have been different for this mom?

7. Describe how she received equitable empathy and respectful care. Who did she receive it from?

CHAPTER 10

Important Terms For Doulas

Here's a helpful alphabetical guide to key terms often used in the doula and childbirth community:

Active Labor

The phase of labor where contractions become more regular, stronger, and closer together, leading to the dilation of the cervix from 6 cm to full dilation at 10 cm.

Advocacy

The process of supporting and empowering a pregnant person to make informed decisions about their care, including speaking up for their rights and preferences during labor and delivery.

Balloon Catheter

A medical device used to mechanically dilate the cervix during induction by placing a balloon into the cervix and inflating it with saline.

Birth Plan

A written document that outlines a pregnant person's preferences for labor, delivery, and postpartum care, including medical interventions, pain management, and who will be present during the birth.

Cervical Effacement

The thinning and shortening of the cervix in preparation for labor, measured in percentages, with 100% being fully effaced.

Cervical Dilation

The opening of the cervix during labor, measured in centimeters from 0 to 10 cm, with 10 cm indicating full dilation and readiness for pushing.

Cesarean Section (C-Section)

A surgical procedure to deliver a baby through incisions in the abdomen and uterus, often recommended when a vaginal delivery isn't possible or safe.

Comfort Measures

Techniques used during labor to ease discomfort, such as breathing exercises, massage, movement, and changing positions.

Contraction

A tightening and releasing of the uterine muscles during labor, helping to dilate the cervix and push the baby down through the birth canal.

Doula

A trained professional who provides emotional, physical, and informational support to a birthing person before, during, and after childbirth.

Epidural

A form of anesthesia commonly used during labor to relieve pain by injecting medication into the epidural space of the spine.

Fetal Station

Refers to the baby's position in the pelvis, measured in relation to the ischial spines. A baby at station 0 is engaged in the pelvis, while positive numbers (+1 to +3) indicate descent into the birth canal.

Hyperemesis Gravidarum

A severe form of morning sickness characterized by excessive nausea and vomiting during pregnancy, often requiring medical treatment and sometimes hospitalization.

Induction

The medical process of stimulating labor, typically through medications like Pitocin or by other means like breaking the water or using a balloon catheter.

Labor Positions

Various body positions (e.g., squatting, hands and knees, side-lying) that can help ease labor pain, improve contractions, and assist in moving the baby down the birth canal.

Oxytocin

A hormone that plays a key role in childbirth, helping to stimulate uterine contractions and promote bonding and milk production post-birth.

Pain Management

The different methods used to relieve labor pain, including breathing techniques, medications (like epidurals), and alternative therapies (e.g., water immersion or hypnobirthing).

Perineum

The area between the vagina and the anus, which stretches during childbirth and may be subject to tearing or an episiotomy during delivery.

Pitocin

A synthetic form of oxytocin used to induce or augment labor by stimulating uterine contractions.

Postpartum

The period after childbirth, typically lasting six weeks, during which the birthing person's body adjusts to non-pregnancy, and physical, emotional, and mental changes occur.

Skin-to-Skin Contact

The practice of placing a newborn directly on the mother's chest or abdomen immediately after birth to promote bonding, breastfeeding, and regulate the baby's temperature.

Transition

The last phase of active labor before pushing, characterized by intense contractions as the cervix dilates from 8 to 10 cm.

Unmedicated Birth

A birth where no pain-relief medications (such as epidurals or narcotics) are used, relying on natural methods for managing labor discomfort.

This list provides an overview of the key terms related to labor and delivery that both doulas and clients should understand. Each term is significant in preparing for childbirth and navigating the birth experience.

CHAPTER 12

Scope of Practice

By Dr. Candace Kelly & Felicia Francis-Edwards

Excerpt From **Nurturing Equity Minded Healthcare Providers**

Below you will find a 12-step list outlining the scope of practice for a doula, which encompasses the various roles and responsibilities they undertake to support birthing individuals and families:

12-Step Scope of Practice for a Doula

1. **Emotional Support:** Provide continuous emotional and physical support to the birthing person before, during, and after labor, helping to reduce anxiety and fear.

2. **Educational Resources:** Offer information about pregnancy, childbirth, and postpartum recovery, helping clients make informed decisions about their care options.

3. **Birth Plan Assistance:** Collaborate with clients to create a personalized birth plan, discussing preferences for labor, delivery, and postpartum care.

4. **Comfort Measures:** Teach and assist with non-pharmacological comfort measures, such as breathing techniques, relaxation exercises, and various labor positions.

5. **Advocacy:** Act as an advocate for the birthing person, facilitating communication between them and the medical team, and ensuring their preferences are respected.

6. **Physical Support:** Provide physical support during labor, such as helping with positioning, massage, counter-pressure, and other techniques to alleviate discomfort.

7. **Continuous Presence:** Remain with the birthing person throughout labor and delivery, offering consistent support and reassurance.

8. **Postpartum Support:** Provide postpartum support, including assistance with infant care, breastfeeding education, and emotional support for the new parents.

9. **Resource Referrals:** Connect clients with additional resources and professionals, such as lactation consultants, parenting classes, and mental health support.

10. **Cultural Sensitivity:** Respect and accommodate the diverse cultural, spiritual, and personal beliefs of clients in their birthing practices.

11. **Collaboration with Healthcare Providers:** Work collaboratively with the healthcare team, maintaining clear communication and understanding the roles of each member.

12. **Professional Development:** Engage in ongoing education and training to stay updated on best practices, research, and advancements in maternal health and doula care.

This scope of practice emphasizes the doula's role as a supportive companion and educator, advocating for the birthing person's needs and preferences while promoting a positive and empowering birth experience. Remember to bring your Empathic self to their care, every time.

CHAPTER 13

Nine Pillars of Entering the Sacred Space

By Dr. Candace Kelly & Felicia Francis-Edwards

Excerpt from **Nurturing Equity Minded Healthcare Providers**

Every Doula must embrace the Nine Pillars of entering the sacred space of a client. Here are nine ways to enter a client's space as a doula, each defined to emphasize the importance of creating a supportive and trusting environment:

1. HUMILITY

Definition: Approach each client with a sense of humility, recognizing that every birthing experience is unique and that you are there to support them, not impose your beliefs or experiences.

Application: Listen actively to your client's needs, acknowledging their expertise in their own bodies and experiences. This creates a safe space where they feel valued and heard.

2. CURIOSITY

Definition: Cultivate a genuine sense of curiosity about your client's individual needs, preferences, and experiences.

Application: Ask open-ended questions to better understand their desires for labor and delivery. This encourages them to share their thoughts and feelings, helping you tailor your support to their specific situation.

3. RESPECT

Definition: Show deep respect for your client's choices, values, and cultural beliefs, acknowledging their autonomy throughout the birthing process.

Application: Validate their feelings and decisions without judgment, ensuring they feel empowered to make informed choices about their care and experience.

4. ADVOCACY

Definition: Advocacy involves supporting and empowering the birthing person in expressing their preferences, desires, and rights within the healthcare system.

Application: Be a voice for the birthing person's preferences, desires, and needs. Educate them on their options and rights within the healthcare system, empowering them to make informed decisions. During labor, communicate effectively with the medical team, ensuring the birthing person's wishes are clearly expressed and respected.

5. GENTLENESS

Definition: Approach your clients and their situation with gentleness, both in your demeanor and your actions.

Application: Use a calm and soothing voice, gentle touch, and mindful movements to create a peaceful atmosphere. This helps to ease tension and anxiety, allowing clients to feel more relaxed and supported.

6. DIGNITY

Definition: Treat every client with dignity, recognizing their inherent worth and the importance of their experience.

Application: Ensure their privacy and comfort, respect their boundaries, and address them with kindness and compassion. This helps to foster trust and rapport, making clients feel valued and respected.

7. EDUCATION

Definition: Provide education and information to empower clients in their decision-making process, fostering a sense of confidence and understanding.

Application: Share evidence-based information about pregnancy, labor, and postpartum care while respecting their individual choices. Encourage questions and discussions to ensure they feel informed and involved in their care.

8. ACTIVE LISTENING

Definition: Engage in active listening, giving full attention to your clients and showing empathy towards their feelings and concerns.

Application: Use verbal affirmations and non-verbal cues (like nodding and maintaining eye contact) to show that you are fully present. Reflect back what they say to confirm understanding, which helps clients feel validated and heard.

9. TRUST

Definition: Build a foundation of trust with your clients by being reliable, honest, and transparent in your communication.

Application: Establish clear boundaries and follow through on commitments, ensuring clients feel secure in your presence. Encourage open dialogue, reinforcing that their feelings and choices are respected and valued.

By incorporating these nine principles—Humility, Curiosity, Respect, Advocacy, Gentleness, Dignity, Education, Active Listening, and Trust—doulas can effectively enter and support their clients' spaces, fostering a positive and empowering environment that enhances the birthing experience.

CHAPTER 14

Timeliness

By Dr. Candace Kelly & Felicia Francis-Edwards

Excerpt from **Nurturing Equity Minded Healthcare Providers**

Critically important to showing up in the sacred space as a doula is a focus on timeliness. This is essential for creating a supportive and empowering environment for the birthing person. Here are some key practices to ensure you embody this principle effectively:

1. PREPARATION BEFORE THE BIRTH

Know the Due Date: Keep track of the estimated due date and have a plan in place to be available around that time.

Stay Informed: Maintain communication with the birthing person and their support team to understand any signs of labor onset, preferences, or concerns.

Pack Your Bag Early: Have your doula bag ready with essentials like comfort items, educational materials, and tools to support the birthing process, ensuring you can leave quickly when needed.

2. COMMUNICATION

Establish Clear Expectations: Discuss timelines, preferences, and emergency contacts during your prenatal meetings, ensuring everyone understands your role and availability.

Check In Regularly: Maintain open lines of communication with the birthing person, providing updates and reassurance as the due date approaches.

3. TIMING YOUR ARRIVAL

Arrive at the Right Moment: Be aware of the stages of labor and know when to arrive. For early labor, check in frequently and assess if you need to be there, balancing your presence with their need for privacy.

Use Your Intuition: Trust your instincts about when the birthing person might need you most, being sensitive to their energy and needs.

4. BEING PRESENT IN THE MOMENT

Mindfulness Practices: Ground yourself through mindfulness techniques to remain fully present and focused when you arrive, enhancing your ability to support the birthing person.

Adaptability: Be prepared for changes in plans or timing, maintaining a calm demeanor to help the birthing person feel secure and supported.

5. AFTER THE BIRTH

Stay for Support: Offer continued support in the immediate postpartum period, assisting with breastfeeding, bonding, and the transition into parenthood as needed.

Debrief: After the birth, take time to discuss the experience with the birthing person and their partner, allowing them to share their feelings and thoughts, reinforcing the sacredness of their journey.

6. REFLECTION AND GROWTH

Postpartum Check-Ins: Follow up after the birth to see how they are doing, reinforcing your ongoing support and connection.

Learn from Each Experience: Reflect on each birth experience to improve your timeliness and presence for future clients.

Conclusion

By prioritizing timeliness and presence, you create a sacred space for the birthing person, allowing them to feel safe, supported, and empowered throughout their journey. Your role as a doula is to honor the unique experience of each birth while being adaptable to the needs of the birthing person.

CHAPTER 15

Collaborating with Hospitals and BirthCare Centers

By Dr. Candace Kelly & Felicia Francis-Edwards

Excerpt from **Nurturing Equity Minded Healthcare Providers**

A Doula's 10-step guideline on how to effectively partner with a medical team while honoring their own respective boundaries:

10-Step Guideline for Doulas Partnering with a Medical Team

1. **Understand Your Role:** Clearly define your role as a doula. Understand that you are there to provide emotional, physical, and informational support to the birthing person, not to provide medical care or intervene in clinical decisions.

2. **Establish Communication:** Open lines of communication with the medical team before labor begins. Introduce yourself and explain your role to ensure everyone is on the same page regarding your involvement.

3. **Respect Medical Protocols:** Familiarize yourself with the hospital or birthing center's policies and procedures. Respect the medical team's protocols and work within their framework while advocating for the client's preferences.

4. **Build Collaborative Relationships:** Foster positive relationships with healthcare providers. Show appreciation for their work, and be respectful and cooperative, which can help create a collaborative environment.

5. **Maintain Professional Boundaries:** Clearly define your boundaries as a doula. Communicate these boundaries to both the client and the medical team to ensure everyone understands your role and limitations.

6. **Advocate, Don't Interfere:** Advocate for the birthing person's wishes and preferences respectfully. Use effective communication skills to express their desires without undermining the medical team's authority or decisions.

7. **Stay Calm and Positive:** Maintain a calm and positive demeanor, especially during stressful situations. This helps to create a supportive environment for both the client and the medical team.

8. **Document Important Information:** Keep a record of the client's preferences, any important discussions with the medical team, and any significant changes during labor. This documentation can help facilitate communication and ensure continuity of care.

9. **Encourage Teamwork:** Foster a spirit of teamwork among the medical staff and the client. Encourage the client to express their feelings and concerns to the healthcare team, creating an environment of mutual respect.

10. **Reflect and Debrief:** After the birth, take time to reflect on the experience. If possible, have a debriefing session with the medical team to discuss what went well and what could be improved. This not only fosters relationships but also enhances future collaborations.

When following these guidelines, doulas can effectively partner with medical teams while honoring their boundaries and providing the best possible support for the birthing person.

ABOUT THE AUTHOR

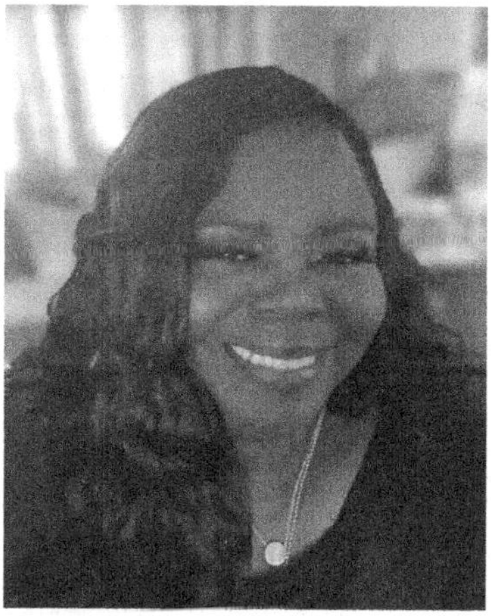

Felicia Francis-Edwards CLES, CD

Felicia is an empathetic birthing professional with over 30 years of experience, dedicated to supporting people of color, specifically African American women, in achieving safe births. She began her career at the Watts Health Foundation, where she provided doula support, case management, and health education for over 16 years. Fluent in English and some Spanish, she educated pregnant parents on childbirth, lactation, and infant care.

After her time at Watts, Felicia transitioned to Youth and Family Services and the CAL-LEARN program, advocating for 30 clients and helping them access critical resources. She completed her Doula training at DONA (Doula of North America) in 2012 and continued her work through Healthnet's Doula program and the AAIM Doula Pilot. Throughout her career, she has supported over 200 births, providing education and advocacy for both pregnant and postpartum clients.

Felicia's vision is to train new doulas and act as a safe mentor, particularly with the start of the medical doula reimbursement initiative. She is committed to achieving equitable maternal and infant care for all people of color, especially Black mothers, to ensure optimal outcomes in safe birthing environments. Felicia also serves as Chief Operating Officer for Still Resilient Redefining Maternal and Infant Health, a nonprofit organization providing equitable empathy education and training to institutions, universities, hospitals, and birth workers.

Felicia firmly believes that every mother deserves equity and postpartum process, and she strives to be an empathic birthing professional and advocate for every mother she serves.

For Booking Doula Training and Speaking Engagements:

Email:
Feliciafrancisedwardsgentle@gmail.com

Books available online at:
Amazon.com
Barnes and Noble
Walmart

Made in the USA
Las Vegas, NV
03 August 2025

25758276R00049